EAT WELL, LIVE WELL COOKBOOK

Balanced Eating Techniques for Fat-Burning, Heal Your Metabolism And Boost Longevity.

MICHAEL JUNIOR

Copyright©2023 Michael Junior

TABLE OF CONTENT

INTRODUCTION

The quest of a balanced and healthful lifestyle has never been more important in a world abounding with gastronomic options.

The "Eat Well, Live Well Cookbook" is more than simply a recipe collection; it's a culinary journey that acknowledges the fundamental link between the food we eat and the energy we nurture.

Within these pages, you'll find a variety of painstakingly produced meals that go beyond ordinary nourishment, urging you to experience the harmonic balance of flavors, textures, and healthful ingredients.

Our approach goes beyond the concept of restricted diets, with the goal of redefining how we view and experience food. Each meal exemplifies the concept that eating healthily is a celebration, not a sacrifice—a celebration of brilliant colors, rich scents, and the innate richness that nature gives.

This cookbook is your companion on the way to health, vigor, and the delight that comes with a well-balanced meal, whether you are an avid home cook or a newbie to the world of culinary inquiry.

Allow the "Eat Well, Live Well Cookbook" to be your guide as you embrace a lifestyle in which every meal is an occasion to indulge in tastes that excite the tongue and nourish the body.

May the recipes in these pages inspire a greater appreciation for the art of eating well as you begin on this culinary adventure, paving the path for a life where health and pleasure live together.

Greek Yogurt Parfait with Nuts and Berries

Scenario:

Imagine waking up to a bright and energizing morning. You're ready to kick-start your day with a delicious and nutritious breakfast that not only satisfies your taste buds but also provides a burst of vitamins, antioxidants, and energy.

This Greek Yogurt Parfait with Nuts and Berries is the perfect blend of creamy yogurt, crunchy nuts, and vibrant berries, making every spoonful a delightful and healthy experience.

Ingredients:

- 1 cup Greek yogurt (unsweetened)
- 1/2 cup mixed berries (strawberries, blueberries, raspberries)
- 1/4 cup granola (choose a low-sugar or homemade option)
- 2 tablespoons mixed nuts (almonds, walnuts, or your favorites)
- 1 tablespoon honey (optional, for drizzling)
- Fresh mint leaves for garnish (optional)

Preparation:
1. **Layer the Base:** Start by spooning a layer of Greek yogurt into a glass or a bowl. Ensure the yogurt is evenly spread at the bottom.

2. **Add Berries:** Sprinkle a handful of mixed berries over the yogurt layer. This adds natural sweetness, fiber, and a pop of color.

3. **Sprinkle Granola:** Evenly distribute granola on top of the berries. The granola adds a satisfying crunch and complex carbohydrates for lasting energy.

4. **Nuts Galore:** Sprinkle a mix of your favorite nuts over the granola. Nuts provide healthy fats, protein, and an additional crunch.

5. **Repeat Layers:** Repeat the layering process until you reach the top of the glass, finishing with a sprinkle of berries and nuts.

6. **Drizzle Honey (Optional):** For a touch of sweetness, drizzle honey over the top. This step is optional, especially if you prefer a less sweet parfait.

7. **Garnish with Mint (Optional):** For a refreshing finish, garnish your parfait with a few fresh mint leaves.

Benefits:
1. **Protein Boost:** Greek yogurt is rich in protein, promoting muscle health and keeping you full throughout the morning.

2. **Antioxidant Powerhouse:** Berries are packed with antioxidants, helping to combat oxidative stress and support overall health.

3. **Heart-Healthy Nuts:** Nuts provide heart-healthy fats, fiber, and essential nutrients that contribute to cardiovascular well-being.

4. **Energy from Granola:** The granola supplies complex carbohydrates, offering a sustained release of energy.

5. **Bone Health:** Greek yogurt is a good source of calcium and contributes to maintaining strong and healthy bones.

Application:
- **Breakfast Delight:** Enjoy this parfait as a wholesome breakfast that sets a positive tone for the day.

- **Snack Attack:** Need a satisfying snack? Grab a smaller portion for a nutritious and delicious snack between meals.

- **Post-Workout Refuel:** The combination of protein, carbs, and healthy fats makes this parfait an excellent choice for post-exercise recovery.

Avocado and Black Bean Salad

Scenario:
Picture a warm summer afternoon, and you're craving a refreshing and nutritious meal. The Avocado and Black Bean Salad is a vibrant and satisfying option that combines the creaminess of ripe avocados with the protein-packed goodness of black beans.

This salad not only tantalizes your taste buds but also provides a healthy dose of essential nutrients, making it a perfect choice for a light lunch or a side dish at a picnic.

Ingredients:
- 2 ripe avocados, diced
- 1 can (15 oz) black beans, drained and rinsed
- 1 cup corn kernels (fresh, canned, or frozen)
- 1/2 red onion, finely chopped
- 1 cup cherry tomatoes, halved
- Fresh cilantro, chopped (to taste)
- 1 lime, juiced
- 2 tablespoons olive oil
- Salt and pepper to taste

Preparation:
1. **Prepare Ingredients:** Dice the ripe avocados, chop the red onion and cilantro, and halve the cherry tomatoes.

2. **Combine Ingredients:** In a large mixing bowl, combine the diced avocados, black beans, corn, red onion, cherry tomatoes, and chopped cilantro.

3. **Make the Dressing:** In a small bowl, whisk together lime juice, olive oil, salt, and pepper. Adjust the seasoning to taste.

4. **Toss and Dress:** Pour the dressing over the salad ingredients and gently toss until everything is well coated.

5. **Chill (Optional):** For enhanced flavors, refrigerate the salad for about 30 minutes before serving.

6. **Serve:** Garnish with extra cilantro if desired and serve chilled or at room temperature.

Benefits:
1. **Nutrient-Rich:** Avocados provide healthy monounsaturated fats and an array of vitamins, while black beans

contribute protein, fiber, and essential minerals.

2. **Antioxidant Boost:** The variety of vegetables in this salad, particularly the tomatoes and cilantro, add antioxidants that support overall health.

3. **Heart Health:** The combination of avocados and olive oil contributes to heart-healthy fats, promoting cardiovascular well-being.

4. **Digestive Health:** Black beans are a good source of fiber, aiding in digestion and promoting a healthy gut.

5. **Vitamin C:** Lime juice not only adds zesty flavor but also provides a dose of vitamin C, which supports the immune system.

Application:
- **Lunchtime Delight:** Enjoy a generous portion of this salad as a light and satisfying lunch.

- **Picnic Perfection:** Pack this salad in a container for a refreshing and portable dish for your next picnic or outdoor gathering.

- **Side Dish Extravaganza:** Serve as a vibrant side dish alongside grilled chicken, fish, or your favorite protein for a well-rounded meal.

Mushroom and Spinach Stuffed Bell Peppers

Scenario:

Imagine a cozy evening at home, where the aroma of roasted bell peppers filled with a savory mixture of mushrooms and spinach wafts through the kitchen.

These Mushroom and Spinach Stuffed Bell Peppers are a comforting and nutritious dish that transforms a regular weekday dinner into a gourmet experience. Packed with earthy flavors and wholesome ingredients, this recipe is a delightful way to elevate your evening meal.

Ingredients:

- 4 large bell peppers, halved and seeds removed
- 2 cups mushrooms, finely chopped
- 2 cups fresh spinach, chopped
- 1 cup cooked quinoa or rice
- 1 onion, finely chopped
- 2 cloves garlic, minced
- 1 cup shredded mozzarella or feta cheese
- 2 tablespoons olive oil
- 1 teaspoon dried oregano
- Salt and pepper to taste
- Fresh parsley for garnish (optional)

Preparation:

1. **Preheat the Oven:** Preheat your oven to 375°F (190°C).

2. **Prepare Bell Peppers:** Cut the bell peppers in half lengthwise, removing seeds and membranes. Place them in a baking dish.

3. **Sauté Vegetables:** In a skillet, heat olive oil over medium heat. Add onions and garlic, sauté until softened. Add chopped mushrooms and cook until they release their moisture. Stir in chopped spinach and cook until wilted.

4. **Combine Ingredients:** In a large mixing bowl, combine the sautéed vegetables, cooked quinoa or rice, and half of the shredded cheese. Season with oregano, salt, and pepper. Mix well.

5. **Stuff the Peppers:** Generously stuff each bell pepper half with the mixture. Top with the remaining shredded cheese.

6. **Bake:** Cover the baking dish with aluminum foil and bake in the preheated oven for 25-30 minutes, or until the peppers are tender.

7. **Broil (Optional):** If you prefer a golden-brown cheesy top, uncover the dish and broil for an additional 2-3 minutes until the cheese is bubbly and lightly browned.

8. **Garnish and Serve:** Remove from the oven, garnish with fresh parsley if desired, and serve warm.

Benefits:
1. **Vegetarian Protein:** This dish provides a hearty dose of plant-based protein from quinoa or rice, making it a satisfying meatless option.

2. **Nutrient-Rich Veggies:** Mushrooms and spinach are rich in vitamins, minerals, and antioxidants, promoting overall health.

3. **Fiber Boost:** Bell peppers are a good source of dietary fiber, supporting digestion and satiety.

4. **Calcium and Protein:** Cheese adds calcium and additional protein to the dish, contributing to bone health and muscle maintenance.

5. **Low-Calorie Option:** Stuffed bell peppers are a flavorful and low-calorie

alternative, making them suitable for those watching their calorie intake.

Application:
- **Weeknight Dinner Delight:** Enjoy these stuffed bell peppers as a wholesome and delicious weeknight dinner.

- **Meal Prep Magic:** Prepare a batch on the weekend for easy and healthy lunches throughout the week.

- **Party Pleaser:** Serve as an elegant appetizer or side dish at gatherings and impress your guests with the rich flavors and vibrant presentation.

These Mushroom and Spinach Stuffed Bell Peppers are a culinary masterpiece that turns a simple vegetable into a gourmet experience.

With its nutritious ingredients and savory taste, this dish is sure to become a household favorite.

Baked Cod with Herbs and Lemon

Scenario:

Imagine a light, flavorful dinner that transports you to the shores of the Mediterranean. The Baked Cod with Herbs and Lemon is a dish that not only tantalizes your taste buds but also provides a healthy dose of omega-3 fatty acids and essential nutrients.

As the aroma of fresh herbs and zesty lemon fills your kitchen, you'll anticipate savoring a delicious and wholesome meal that is both easy to prepare and impressive.

Ingredients:

- 4 cod fillets (about 6 oz each)
- 2 tablespoons olive oil
- 2 cloves garlic, minced
- 1 tablespoon fresh parsley, chopped
- 1 tablespoon fresh dill, chopped
- 1 tablespoon fresh thyme leaves
- Zest of one lemon
- Juice of one lemon
- Salt and pepper to taste
- Lemon slices for garnish

Preparation:

1. **Preheat the Oven:** Preheat your oven to 400°F (200°C).

2. **Prepare Cod Fillets:** Pat the cod fillets dry with paper towels. Place them in a baking dish lined with parchment paper or lightly greased.

3. **Herb Infusion:** In a small bowl, mix together olive oil, minced garlic, chopped parsley, dill, thyme, lemon zest, lemon juice, salt, and pepper.

4. **Coat Cod Fillets:** Brush the cod fillets generously with the herb and lemon mixture, ensuring they are well coated on both sides.

5. **Bake:** Bake in the preheated oven for 15-20 minutes or until the cod is opaque and flakes easily with a fork.

6. **Broil (Optional):** For a golden finish, you can broil the cod for an additional 2-3 minutes, keeping a close eye to prevent burning.

7. **Garnish and Serve:** Remove from the oven, garnish with additional fresh herbs and lemon slices, and serve immediately.

Benefits:

1. **Omega-3 Fatty Acids:** Cod is a rich source of omega-3 fatty acids, which are essential for heart health, brain function, and reducing inflammation.

2. **Herb and Citrus Goodness:** Fresh herbs like parsley, dill, and thyme not only add flavor but also provide antioxidants and essential nutrients. Lemon adds a zesty kick and vitamin C.

3. **Lean Protein:** Cod is a lean protein, making this dish a healthy option for those aiming to reduce saturated fat intake while still enjoying a satisfying meal.

4. **Heart-Healthy Olive Oil:** Olive oil contributes heart-healthy monounsaturated fats to the dish.

5. **Low-Calorie Option:** Baked cod is a flavorful and low-calorie choice, making it suitable for those watching their calorie intake.

Application:

- **Weeknight Elegance:** Serve this baked cod on a weeknight when you want a quick and elegant dinner without much fuss.

- **Dinner Party Delight:** Impress your guests with this sophisticated yet easy-to-make dish at your next dinner party.

- **Healthy Living Staple:** Make this recipe a regular part of your repertoire for a delicious and health-conscious meal option.

The Baked Cod with Herbs and Lemon is a celebration of fresh, wholesome ingredients that come together to create a dish that is both nourishing and delightful.

Enjoy the taste of the Mediterranean in the comfort of your own home.

Cabbage and Apple Slaw

Scenario:

Imagine a crisp and refreshing side dish that adds a burst of color and flavor to your table. The Cabbage and Apple Slaw is a delightful combination of crunchy cabbage and sweet, tangy apples, all brought together with a light and zesty dressing.

Whether served at a picnic, barbecue, or alongside your favorite protein, this slaw is a versatile and healthy addition to any meal, bringing a perfect balance of textures and tastes.

Ingredients:

- 1/2 head of green cabbage, finely shredded
- 2 apples (crisp varieties like Granny Smith or Honeycrisp), julienned
- 1/2 cup Greek yogurt
- 2 tablespoons mayonnaise
- 1 tablespoon Dijon mustard
- 1 tablespoon honey
- 1 tablespoon apple cider vinegar
- Salt and pepper to taste
- 1/4 cup raisins or dried cranberries (optional)

- Chopped fresh parsley for garnish (optional)

Preparation:
1. **Prepare Vegetables and Fruit:** Finely shred the green cabbage and julienne the apples. Place them in a large mixing bowl.

2. **Make Dressing:** In a small bowl, whisk together Greek yogurt, mayonnaise, Dijon mustard, honey, apple cider vinegar, salt, and pepper until well combined.

3. **Combine Ingredients:** Pour the dressing over the shredded cabbage and apples. Toss the ingredients together until the slaw is evenly coated with the dressing.

4. **Optional Additions:** If desired, add raisins or dried cranberries for a sweet touch and extra texture.

5. **Chill (Optional):** For enhanced flavors, refrigerate the slaw for about 30 minutes before serving.

6. **Garnish and Serve:** Garnish with chopped fresh parsley if desired and serve chilled or at room temperature.

Benefits:

1. **Vitamin C Boost:** Cabbage and apples are rich in vitamin C, providing an immune system boost and promoting healthy skin.

2. **Fiber-Rich:** Both cabbage and apples are excellent sources of dietary fiber, aiding in digestion and promoting a feeling of fullness.

3. **Probiotics from Yogurt:** Greek yogurt in the dressing contributes probiotics, supporting gut health.

4. **Antioxidant Properties:** The combination of cabbage and apples offers a variety of antioxidants, helping combat oxidative stress.

5. **Light and Nutritious:** The dressing uses a combination of Greek yogurt and a touch of mayonnaise, providing a lighter alternative to traditional coleslaw dressings.

Application:

- **Picnic Perfect:** Pack this slaw for a picnic or outdoor gathering. It pairs well with grilled meats or sandwiches.

- **Burger Buddy:** Serve as a refreshing side with burgers or barbecue dishes.

- **Lunchtime Delight:** Enjoy a bowl of Cabbage and Apple Slaw on its own or as a side with your favorite protein for a light and nutritious lunch.

The Cabbage and Apple Slaw is a versatile and vibrant dish that brings together the crispness of cabbage and the sweetness of apples, creating a perfect harmony of flavors.

Add this slaw to your repertoire for a fresh and health-conscious side option.

Grilled Chicken and Asparagus

Scenario:
Picture a warm summer evening, the sun setting, and the enticing aroma of grilled chicken and asparagus wafting through the air. The Grilled Chicken and Asparagus recipe is a simple yet elegant dish that brings the smoky flavors of the grill to your dinner table.

Whether you're hosting a backyard barbecue or looking for a quick and wholesome weeknight meal, this recipe is sure to become a family favorite.

Ingredients:
- 4 boneless, skinless chicken breasts
- 1 bunch of fresh asparagus, trimmed
- 2 tablespoons olive oil
- 3 cloves garlic, minced
- 1 teaspoon dried oregano
- 1 teaspoon paprika
- Salt and pepper to taste
- Zest and juice of one lemon
- Fresh parsley for garnish (optional)

Preparation:
1. **Preheat the Grill:** Preheat your grill to medium-high heat.

2. **Prepare Chicken:** In a bowl, mix olive oil, minced garlic, dried oregano, paprika, salt, pepper, and the zest of one lemon. Coat the chicken breasts with this mixture, ensuring they are well-seasoned.

3. **Grill Chicken:** Place the seasoned chicken breasts on the preheated grill. Grill for about 6-8 minutes per side or until the internal temperature reaches 165°F (74°C) and the chicken is cooked through.

4. **Prepare Asparagus:** While the chicken is grilling, toss the trimmed asparagus with a drizzle of olive oil, salt, and pepper.

5. **Grill Asparagus:** Add the asparagus to the grill during the last 3-4 minutes of cooking the chicken. Grill until the asparagus is tender-crisp with a slight char.

6. **Lemon Finish:** Squeeze the juice of one lemon over the grilled chicken and asparagus just before removing them from the grill.

7. **Garnish and Serve:** Garnish with fresh parsley if desired and serve immediately.

Benefits:

1. **Lean Protein:** Chicken breasts provide a lean source of protein, essential for muscle maintenance and repair.

2. **Nutrient-Rich Asparagus:** Asparagus is a good source of vitamins A, C, and K, as well as folate and fiber.

3. **Heart-Healthy Olive Oil:** The olive oil used in the marinade contributes heart-healthy monounsaturated fats.

4. **Low-Calorie Option:** Grilled chicken and asparagus is a flavorful and low-calorie choice, making it suitable for those watching their calorie intake.

5. **Lemon Zest:** The addition of lemon zest and juice not only enhances flavor but also provides vitamin C and a burst of freshness.

Application:

- **Backyard Barbecue:** Impress your guests with this simple and delicious grilled dish at your next barbecue gathering.

- **Quick Weeknight Dinner:** This recipe is perfect for a quick and satisfying

weeknight dinner, providing a balanced meal.
- **Meal Prep Magic:** Grill extra chicken and asparagus to use in salads, wraps, or bowls throughout the week.

The Grilled Chicken and Asparagus recipe offers a perfect balance of flavors and textures, showcasing the simplicity and versatility of grilled ingredients.

Whether you're a grilling enthusiast or a novice, this dish is a fantastic addition to your culinary repertoire.

Spaghetti Squash with Pesto and Cherry Tomatoes

Scenario:
Envision a light and flavorful dinner that not only satisfies your pasta cravings but also introduces a healthy twist. Spaghetti Squash with Pesto and Cherry Tomatoes is a vibrant and nutritious alternative to traditional pasta dishes.

As you twirl the delicate strands of spaghetti squash coated in fresh pesto and adorned with sweet cherry tomatoes, you'll savor a guilt-free and delicious meal that's perfect for a cozy evening at home.

Ingredients:
- 1 medium-sized spaghetti squash
- 1 cup cherry tomatoes, halved
- 1/2 cup fresh basil leaves
- 1/4 cup pine nuts
- 1/2 cup grated Parmesan cheese
- 2 cloves garlic, peeled
- 1/2 cup extra-virgin olive oil
- Salt and pepper to taste
- Red pepper flakes for a hint of heat (optional)
- Fresh basil for garnish (optional)

Preparation:

1. **Preheat the Oven:** Preheat your oven to 375°F (190°C).

2. **Prepare the Spaghetti Squash:** Cut the spaghetti squash in half lengthwise. Scoop out the seeds. Place the halves, cut side down, on a baking sheet. Bake for 40-45 minutes or until the flesh is tender.

3. **Make the Pesto:** While the squash is baking, prepare the pesto. In a food processor, combine fresh basil, pine nuts, Parmesan cheese, garlic, salt, and pepper. Pulse until coarsely chopped. With the processor running, slowly stream in the olive oil until a smooth pesto forms.

4. **Scrape the Squash:** Once the spaghetti squash is cooked, use a fork to scrape the flesh into strands. Place the strands in a large mixing bowl.

5. **Toss with Pesto:** Add the prepared pesto to the spaghetti squash strands. Toss until the squash is evenly coated with the pesto.

6. **Add Cherry Tomatoes:** Gently fold in the halved cherry tomatoes, ensuring they are distributed throughout the dish.

7. **Adjust Seasoning:** Taste and adjust the seasoning with salt, pepper, and red pepper flakes if desired.

8. **Garnish and Serve:** Garnish with fresh basil if desired. Serve warm, and enjoy your delightful spaghetti squash creation.

Benefits:
1. **Low-Calorie Alternative:** Spaghetti squash is a low-calorie, nutrient-rich alternative to traditional pasta, making it suitable for those seeking a lighter option.

2. **Healthy Fats from Pesto:** Olive oil and pine nuts in the pesto contribute heart-healthy monounsaturated fats.

3. **Vitamins and Minerals:** Cherry tomatoes provide a burst of vitamins A and C, as well as essential minerals.

4. **Nutrient-Packed Basil:** Fresh basil is rich in antioxidants, vitamins, and minerals.

5. **Versatile and Gluten-Free:** This dish is gluten-free and accommodates various dietary preferences.

Application:
- **Weeknight Delight:** Enjoy this dish as a quick and healthy weeknight dinner that comes together effortlessly.

- **Lunchtime Elegance:** Pack leftovers for a sophisticated and nutritious lunch at work or school.

- **Dinner Party Hit:** Impress your guests with this elegant yet simple dish at your next dinner gathering.

Spaghetti Squash with Pesto and Cherry Tomatoes is a celebration of fresh, vibrant flavors that redefine the concept of comfort food.

As you savor each forkful, you'll appreciate the health-conscious twist on a classic dish.

Lentil and Vegetable Stew

Scenario:

Imagine a cozy evening, perhaps with rain tapping gently on the windows. The scent of simmering lentils, vegetables, and aromatic spices fills your kitchen.

Lentil and Vegetable Stew is a comforting and nourishing dish that warms your soul and satisfies your appetite. Whether you're looking for a hearty meal after a long day or a plant-based option for a family dinner, this stew provides a flavorful and wholesome experience.

Ingredients:

- 1 cup dried green or brown lentils, rinsed and drained
- 1 large onion, finely chopped
- 2 carrots, peeled and diced
- 2 celery stalks, diced
- 3 cloves garlic, minced
- 1 can (14 oz) diced tomatoes
- 4 cups vegetable broth
- 1 teaspoon ground cumin
- 1 teaspoon smoked paprika
- 1/2 teaspoon ground coriander
- 1/2 teaspoon dried thyme
- Salt and pepper to taste
- 2 cups chopped kale or spinach

- 2 tablespoons olive oil
- Fresh parsley for garnish (optional)
- Crusty bread for serving

Preparation:
1. **Sauté Aromatics:** In a large pot, heat olive oil over medium heat. Add chopped onion, carrots, celery, and garlic. Sauté until the vegetables are softened, about 5-7 minutes.

2. **Add Lentils:** Stir in the rinsed lentils, ensuring they are well coated with the sautéed vegetables.

3. **Spice It Up:** Add ground cumin, smoked paprika, ground coriander, dried thyme, salt, and pepper. Stir well to combine and toast the spices for about 1-2 minutes.

4. **Pour in Broth and Tomatoes:** Pour in the vegetable broth and diced tomatoes (with their juices). Bring the mixture to a boil, then reduce the heat to low and let it simmer, covered, for 25-30 minutes or until the lentils are tender.

5. **Add Greens:** Stir in the chopped kale or spinach and cook for an additional 5 minutes until the greens are wilted.

6. **Adjust Seasoning:** Taste and adjust the seasoning, adding more salt and pepper if needed.

7. **Garnish and Serve:** Ladle the stew into bowls, garnish with fresh parsley if desired, and serve with crusty bread.

Benefits:
   1. **Plant-Based Protein:** Lentils are a rich source of plant-based protein, essential for muscle repair and overall health.

   2. **Fiber-Rich:** Lentils and vegetables provide dietary fiber, promoting digestive health and satiety.

   3. **Vitamins and Minerals:** Carrots, celery, and leafy greens contribute essential vitamins and minerals, such as vitamin A, vitamin K, and folate.

   4. **Heart-Healthy Spices:** Cumin, coriander, and thyme not only add depth of flavor but also offer potential heart health benefits.

   5. **Low in Saturated Fat:** This stew is naturally low in saturated fat, making it a heart-healthy option.

Application:

- **Comforting Dinner:** Serve this stew as a comforting and nutritious dinner on chilly evenings.

- **Meal Prep:** Prepare a batch on the weekend for easy and healthy lunches throughout the week.

- **Family-Friendly Option:** Share this wholesome stew with family and friends as a filling and satisfying main course.

Lentil and Vegetable Stew is a celebration of simple, nutritious ingredients that come together to create a nourishing and flavorful meal. It's a reminder that healthy eating can be both satisfying and delicious.

Chia Seed Pudding with Berries

Scenario:
Imagine starting your day with a delightful and nutrient-packed breakfast that feels like a treat. Chia Seed Pudding with Berries is a perfect embodiment of that scenario.

As you spoon into the creamy pudding, the burst of freshness from the vibrant berries complements the subtle sweetness of the chia seeds. This recipe is not only delicious but also a wholesome way to kick-start your morning or enjoy a guilt-free dessert.

Ingredients:
- 1/4 cup chia seeds
- 1 cup unsweetened almond milk (or any milk of your choice)
- 1 tablespoon maple syrup or honey (optional, for sweetness)
- 1/2 teaspoon vanilla extract
- A mix of fresh berries (strawberries, blueberries, raspberries)
- 2 tablespoons sliced almonds or your favorite nuts
- Fresh mint leaves for garnish (optional)

Preparation:

1. **Prepare Chia Seed Mixture:** In a bowl, combine chia seeds, almond milk, maple syrup (if using), and vanilla extract. Whisk well to ensure the chia seeds are evenly distributed.

2. **Let It Set:** Cover the bowl and refrigerate the chia seed mixture for at least 4 hours or overnight. This allows the chia seeds to absorb the liquid and form a pudding-like consistency.

3. **Stir and Adjust:** After the chia seed mixture has set, give it a good stir. If the pudding is too thick, you can add a little more almond milk to achieve your desired consistency.

4. **Layer with Berries:** In serving glasses or bowls, layer the chia seed pudding with a mix of fresh berries.

5. **Top with Nuts:** Sprinkle sliced almonds or your favorite nuts over the berries. This adds a delightful crunch and additional nutrients.

6. **Garnish and Serve:** Garnish with fresh mint leaves if desired. Serve immediately

and enjoy your Chia Seed Pudding with Berries.

Benefits:
1. **Omega-3 Fatty Acids:** Chia seeds are rich in omega-3 fatty acids, supporting heart health and brain function.

2. **Plant-Based Protein:** Chia seeds provide a good source of plant-based protein, helping to keep you full and satisfied.

3. **Dietary Fiber:** Both chia seeds and berries contribute dietary fiber, promoting digestive health and providing a feeling of fullness.

4. **Antioxidant Power:** Berries are packed with antioxidants, which help combat oxidative stress and support overall well-being.

5. **Vitamins and Minerals:** Berries contain essential vitamins and minerals, such as vitamin C and potassium, contributing to a well-rounded nutritional profile.

Application:
- **Breakfast Bliss:** Start your day with a serving of Chia Seed Pudding with Berries for a nutritious and energizing breakfast.

- **Healthy Snack:** Enjoy a smaller portion as a satisfying and healthy snack between meals.

- **Dessert Delight:** Serve this pudding as a guilt-free dessert option at the end of a meal, satisfying your sweet tooth with wholesome ingredients.

Chia Seed Pudding with Berries is a versatile and delightful dish that proves healthy eating can be a delicious experience.

It's a fantastic addition to your culinary repertoire, offering a balance of flavors, textures, and nutritional benefits.

Roasted Brussels Sprouts with Balsamic Glaze

Scenario:

Imagine a side dish that transforms humble Brussels sprouts into a caramelized, savory delight. The Roasted Brussels Sprouts with Balsamic Glaze recipe is the perfect embodiment of this scenario.

As you pull the golden-brown sprouts from the oven and drizzle them with a luscious balsamic glaze, the enticing aroma fills your kitchen. This dish is not only a testament to the magic of roasting but also a celebration of simple ingredients turned into a flavorful masterpiece.

Ingredients:

- 1 lb Brussels sprouts, trimmed and halved
- 2 tablespoons olive oil
- Salt and pepper to taste
- 2 tablespoons balsamic glaze
- 1 tablespoon honey (optional, for added sweetness)
- 1/4 cup grated Parmesan cheese (optional, for garnish)
- Crushed red pepper flakes for a hint of heat (optional)
- Chopped fresh parsley for garnish (optional)

Preparation:

1. **Preheat the Oven:** Preheat your oven to 400°F (200°C).

2. **Prepare Brussels Sprouts:** Trim the Brussels sprouts and cut them in half. Place them on a baking sheet.

3. **Coat with Olive Oil:** Drizzle olive oil over the Brussels sprouts, ensuring they are evenly coated. Season with salt and pepper to taste. Toss to coat them evenly.

4. **Roast:** Roast the Brussels sprouts in the preheated oven for 25-30 minutes or until they are golden brown and crispy on the edges. Shake the pan or toss the sprouts halfway through for even roasting.

5. **Prepare Balsamic Glaze:** While the Brussels sprouts are roasting, heat balsamic glaze in a small saucepan over low heat. If using honey, stir it into the glaze until well combined. Simmer for a few minutes until the glaze thickens slightly.

6. **Drizzle with Glaze:** Once the Brussels sprouts are done roasting, transfer them to a serving dish, and drizzle with the balsamic glaze.

7. **Garnish (Optional):** If desired, garnish with grated Parmesan cheese, crushed red pepper flakes, and chopped fresh parsley for added flavor and presentation.

8. **Serve:** Serve the Roasted Brussels Sprouts with Balsamic Glaze immediately as a flavorful and savory side dish.

Benefits:
1. **Rich in Nutrients:** Brussels sprouts are a good source of vitamins K and C, fiber, and various antioxidants.

2. **Heart-Healthy Olive Oil:** The use of olive oil provides heart-healthy monounsaturated fats.

3. **Balsamic Glaze Goodness:** Balsamic glaze adds a sweet and tangy flavor along with potential health benefits from antioxidants.

4. **Versatile Garnishes:** Parmesan cheese, red pepper flakes, and fresh parsley not only enhance the taste but also contribute additional nutrients.

Application:

- **Holiday Feast:** Serve this dish as a standout side at your holiday gatherings, adding a touch of elegance to the table.

- **Weeknight Delight:** Enjoy as a quick and delicious side for weeknight dinners, complementing various main courses.

- **Appetizer Upgrade:** Offer these Brussels sprouts as an upscale appetizer for special occasions or gatherings.

Roasted Brussels Sprouts with Balsamic Glaze is a versatile and crowd-pleasing dish that elevates the humble Brussels sprout to new heights.

Whether as a side or a standalone appetizer, this recipe is a surefire way to make Brussels sprouts the star of the show.

Lean Turkey and Black Bean Chili

Scenario:

Imagine a chilly evening, and you're craving a comforting bowl of hearty chili. The Lean Turkey and Black Bean Chili is the perfect solution.

The aroma of simmering spices and the wholesome ingredients fill your kitchen, creating an atmosphere of warmth and anticipation.

As you ladle this flavorful chili into bowls and top it with your favorite garnishes, you know you're about to enjoy a nourishing and satisfying meal.

Ingredients:
- 1 lb lean ground turkey
- 1 onion, diced
- 3 cloves garlic, minced
- 1 bell pepper, diced (any color)
- 1 can (15 oz) black beans, drained and rinsed
- 1 can (14 oz) diced tomatoes, undrained
- 1 cup corn kernels (fresh, canned, or frozen)
- 2 cups low-sodium chicken or vegetable broth
- 1 tablespoon chili powder

- 1 teaspoon ground cumin
- 1/2 teaspoon smoked paprika
- Salt and pepper to taste
- Optional toppings: shredded cheese, diced avocado, chopped green onions, cilantro, lime wedges

Preparation:
1. **Brown the Turkey:** In a large pot over medium heat, brown the lean ground turkey until cooked through. Break it into crumbles with a spoon as it cooks.

2. **Sauté Aromatics:** Add diced onion, minced garlic, and diced bell pepper to the pot. Sauté until the vegetables are softened.

3. **Add Beans and Tomatoes:** Stir in the drained and rinsed black beans, undrained diced tomatoes, and corn kernels.

4. **Season the Chili:** Add chili powder, ground cumin, smoked paprika, salt, and pepper. Mix well to ensure the spices are evenly distributed.

5. **Pour in Broth:** Pour in the low-sodium chicken or vegetable broth, stirring to combine all the ingredients.

6. **Simmer:** Bring the chili to a simmer, then reduce the heat to low. Cover and let it simmer for at least 20-30 minutes to allow the flavors to meld.

7. **Adjust Seasoning:** Taste and adjust the seasoning as needed. Add more salt, pepper, or spices to suit your preference.

8. **Serve:** Ladle the Lean Turkey and Black Bean Chili into bowls. Top with shredded cheese, diced avocado, chopped green onions, cilantro, or a squeeze of lime juice, if desired.

Benefits:
1. **Lean Protein:** Turkey provides lean protein, essential for muscle development and repair.

2. **Fiber-Rich Black Beans:** Black beans contribute dietary fiber, promoting digestive health and providing a feeling of fullness.

3. **Vegetables for Nutrients:** Bell peppers and onions add vitamins and minerals to the chili, enhancing its nutritional profile.

4. **Low-Calorie Option:** Using lean turkey and incorporating plenty of vegetables makes this chili a flavorful yet low-calorie option.

5. **Versatile Toppings:** Toppings like avocado and cilantro not only enhance flavor but also offer additional nutrients and freshness.

Application:
- **Game Day Gathering:** Serve this chili as a crowd-pleasing option for game day gatherings.

- **Meal Prep:** Prepare a batch for meal prep, as it reheats well and can be enjoyed throughout the week.

- **Family Dinner Favorite:** Share this wholesome chili with your family for a comforting and nutritious dinner.

Lean Turkey and Black Bean Chili is a delicious and nutritious twist on a classic comfort food. With its lean protein, fiber-rich beans, and flavorful spices, it's a perfect dish for those seeking a satisfying and health-conscious meal.

Egg White Omelet with Vegetables

Scenario:

Imagine a bright morning with the sun streaming into your kitchen. You crave a nutritious and protein-packed breakfast to kickstart your day. The Egg White Omelet with Vegetables is a perfect solution.

As you sauté vibrant vegetables and whisk egg whites to fluffy perfection, the enticing aroma fills your kitchen. The result is a delicious and healthy omelet, bursting with colors and flavors, ready to energize your morning.

Ingredients:
- 4 egg whites
- 1/4 cup diced bell peppers (any color)
- 1/4 cup diced tomatoes
- 1/4 cup diced onions
- 1/4 cup chopped spinach or kale
- 1 tablespoon olive oil
- Salt and pepper to taste
- Optional toppings: diced avocado, feta cheese, salsa, fresh herbs

Preparation:
1. **Prepare Vegetables:** Heat olive oil in a non-stick skillet over medium heat. Add diced bell peppers, tomatoes, onions, and

chopped spinach or kale. Sauté until the vegetables are softened but still vibrant.

2. **Whisk Egg Whites:** While the vegetables are cooking, whisk the egg whites in a bowl until they become frothy. Season with a pinch of salt and pepper.

3. **Add Egg Whites to Skillet:** Pour the whisked egg whites evenly over the sautéed vegetables in the skillet.

4. **Swirl and Cook:** Using a spatula, gently swirl the mixture around the skillet, allowing the uncooked egg whites to flow to the edges. Cook for 2-3 minutes until the edges start to set.

5. **Fold and Flip:** Once the edges are set, carefully fold one side of the omelet over the vegetables, creating a half-moon shape. If desired, you can flip the omelet to cook the other side briefly.

6. **Serve:** Slide the Egg White Omelet onto a plate, folding it onto itself if necessary.

7. **Add Toppings:** Garnish with diced avocado, crumbled feta cheese, salsa, or fresh herbs for added flavor and texture.

8. **Enjoy Immediately:** Serve the omelet hot and savor the delicious combination of fluffy egg whites and vibrant vegetables.

Benefits:
1. **High-Quality Protein:** Egg whites are rich in high-quality protein, essential for muscle maintenance and repair.

2. **Low in Calories:** Egg white omelets are naturally low in calories, making them a great option for those watching their calorie intake.

3. **Nutrient-Rich Vegetables:** Bell peppers, tomatoes, onions, and leafy greens provide essential vitamins, minerals, and antioxidants.

4. **Heart-Healthy Olive Oil:** The use of olive oil adds heart-healthy monounsaturated fats to the dish.

5. **Customizable Toppings:** Toppings like avocado and feta cheese not only enhance flavor but also contribute healthy fats and additional nutrients.

Application:
- **Morning Boost:** Enjoy this omelet as a protein-packed and nutritious breakfast to start your day on a positive note.
- **Quick Lunch:** Whip up a speedy and healthy lunch by making this omelet with your favorite veggies.

- **Post-Workout Refuel:** Replenish your energy after a workout with a satisfying egg white omelet.

The Egg White Omelet with Vegetables is a versatile and wholesome dish that suits various occasions. Whether you're aiming for a healthy breakfast, a quick lunch, or a post-workout refuel, this omelet provides a delicious and nutritious solution.

Mango-Kale Smoothie

Scenario:
Picture a sunny morning, and you're yearning for a refreshing and nutrient-packed start to your day. The Mango-Kale Smoothie is a vibrant solution.

As you blend together sweet mango, earthy kale, and other wholesome ingredients, the smoothie becomes a burst of tropical flavor. Sipping on this green elixir, you feel invigorated and ready to take on the day, knowing you've nourished your body with a delicious and healthful concoction.

Ingredients:
- 1 cup frozen mango chunks
- 1 cup fresh kale leaves, stems removed
- 1/2 banana
- 1/2 cup Greek yogurt
- 1 tablespoon chia seeds
- 1 tablespoon honey (optional, for added sweetness)
- 1 cup unsweetened almond milk (or any milk of your choice)
- Ice cubes (optional)
- Fresh mint leaves for garnish (optional)

Preparation:
1. **Prepare Ingredients:** Ensure the mango chunks are frozen for a creamy texture. Remove the stems from the kale leaves.

2. **Blending Time:** In a blender, combine the frozen mango chunks, kale leaves, banana, Greek yogurt, chia seeds, honey (if using), and unsweetened almond milk.

3. **Blend Until Smooth:** Blend on high speed until the mixture is smooth and creamy. If desired, add ice cubes for a colder consistency.

4. **Adjust Consistency:** If the smoothie is too thick, add more almond milk, a little at a time, until you reach your desired consistency.

5. **Taste and Adjust:** Taste the smoothie and adjust sweetness by adding more honey if needed.

6. **Serve:** Pour the Mango-Kale Smoothie into a glass. Garnish with fresh mint leaves if desired.

7. **Enjoy Immediately:** Sip and savor the refreshing taste of this nutrient-packed smoothie.

Benefits:

1. **Vitamins and Antioxidants:** Mango and kale provide a wealth of vitamins, including vitamin C and vitamin K, as well as antioxidants that support overall health.

2. **Fiber-Rich:** Kale and chia seeds contribute dietary fiber, promoting digestion and providing a feeling of fullness.

3. **Protein Boost:** Greek yogurt adds a protein boost, essential for muscle maintenance and overall energy.

4. **Healthy Fats:** Chia seeds offer omega-3 fatty acids, providing heart-healthy fats.

5. **Hydration:** Almond milk not only adds creaminess but also contributes to overall hydration.

Application:

- **Breakfast Bliss:** Kickstart your day with this Mango-Kale Smoothie for a nutritious and energizing breakfast.

- **Post-Workout Refuel:** Enjoy this smoothie as a refreshing post-workout drink to replenish nutrients.

- **Snack Attack:** Sip on this smoothie as a healthy and satisfying snack between meals.

The Mango-Kale Smoothie is a delightful and nutritious way to incorporate more fruits and vegetables into your diet. With its sweet and tropical flavor profile, it's an excellent choice for those looking to enjoy a healthful and delicious beverage.

Cauliflower Rice Sushi Rolls

Scenario:

Imagine hosting a sushi night at home, and you want to create a healthier twist on traditional sushi. The Cauliflower Rice Sushi Rolls are the perfect solution.

As you assemble these colorful rolls filled with fresh vegetables and creamy avocado, you're not only indulging in a delicious meal but also enjoying a lighter and low-carb alternative to traditional sushi.

The result is a feast for the senses, where every bite is a celebration of flavors and textures.

Ingredients:

- 1 head cauliflower, riced
- 2 tablespoons rice vinegar
- 1 tablespoon sugar
- 1/2 teaspoon salt
- Nori (seaweed) sheets
- Assorted fillings (e.g., cucumber strips, avocado slices, carrot matchsticks, bell pepper strips, cooked shrimp or crab, etc.)
- Soy sauce and pickled ginger for serving
- Sesame seeds and chopped green onions for garnish (optional)

Preparation:

1. **Prepare Cauliflower Rice:** Grate or process the cauliflower in a food processor to create cauliflower rice.

2. **Cook Cauliflower Rice:** In a large skillet, cook the cauliflower rice over medium heat for 5-7 minutes until it becomes tender. Allow it to cool slightly.

3. **Prepare Seasoning:** In a small bowl, mix rice vinegar, sugar, and salt. Gently fold this mixture into the cooked cauliflower rice. Set aside to cool completely.

4. **Assemble Sushi Rolls:** Place a sheet of nori on a bamboo sushi rolling mat. Wet your hands to prevent sticking, and spread a thin layer of seasoned cauliflower rice over the nori, leaving a small border at the top.

5. **Add Fillings:** Arrange your desired fillings in the center of the rice-covered nori.

6. **Roll Sushi:** Using the bamboo mat, carefully roll the nori and fillings into a

tight cylinder. Seal the edge with a dab of water.

7. **Slice and Serve:** Using a sharp knife, slice the roll into bite-sized pieces. Repeat the process with the remaining ingredients.

8. **Garnish and Serve:** Arrange the Cauliflower Rice Sushi Rolls on a platter. Garnish with sesame seeds and chopped green onions if desired.

9. **Serve with Soy Sauce and Pickled Ginger:** Present the sushi rolls with soy sauce and pickled ginger for dipping.

Benefits:
1. **Low-Carb Alternative:** Cauliflower rice replaces traditional sushi rice, offering a lower-carb option suitable for various dietary preferences.

2. **Vitamins and Minerals:** The assorted vegetable fillings provide a range of vitamins and minerals, contributing to a well-rounded and nutritious meal.

3. **Healthy Fats:** Avocado slices add creamy texture and heart-healthy fats to the rolls.

4. **Protein Options:** Incorporate protein sources like shrimp, crab, or tofu for a satisfying and balanced meal.

5. **Fiber-Rich:** Cauliflower and vegetables contribute dietary fiber, promoting digestive health.

Application:
- **Healthy Sushi Night:** Host a sushi night at home with friends or family, showcasing a healthier version of this beloved dish.

- **Lunchbox Delight:** Pack Cauliflower Rice Sushi Rolls in your lunchbox for a satisfying and nutritious midday meal.

- **Appetizer for Gatherings:** Serve these rolls as an elegant and health-conscious appetizer at parties or gatherings.

Cauliflower Rice Sushi Rolls are a creative and nutritious twist on classic sushi, proving that healthier alternatives can be just as delicious and visually appealing.

This recipe offers a delightful way to enjoy the flavors of sushi while embracing a lighter and veggie-packed option.

Sweet Potato and Chickpea Buddha Bowl

Scenario:
Imagine a nourishing and vibrant dinner scenario where you're savoring a colorful array of wholesome ingredients in a single bowl. The Sweet Potato and Chickpea Buddha Bowl is a celebration of flavors, textures, and nutrition.

As you assemble this bowl filled with roasted sweet potatoes, spiced chickpeas, and an assortment of fresh vegetables, you're creating a satisfying and balanced meal that's as pleasing to the eyes as it is to the palate.

Ingredients:
- 1 large sweet potato, peeled and cubed
- 1 can (15 oz) chickpeas, drained and rinsed
- 2 tablespoons olive oil
- 1 teaspoon ground cumin
- 1 teaspoon smoked paprika
- Salt and pepper to taste
- 2 cups cooked quinoa or brown rice
- 1 cup cherry tomatoes, halved
- 1 cucumber, sliced
- 1 avocado, sliced

- 2 cups mixed greens (e.g., spinach, kale, arugula)
- Tahini dressing or your favorite dressing for drizzling
- Sesame seeds for garnish (optional)
- Lemon wedges for serving

Preparation:
1. **Roast Sweet Potatoes and Chickpeas:** Preheat the oven to 425°F (220°C). In a large bowl, toss the cubed sweet potatoes and chickpeas with olive oil, ground cumin, smoked paprika, salt, and pepper. Spread them on a baking sheet in a single layer and roast for 20-25 minutes or until the sweet potatoes are tender and the chickpeas are crispy.

2. **Prepare Quinoa or Brown Rice:** While the sweet potatoes and chickpeas are roasting, cook quinoa or brown rice according to package instructions.

3. **Assemble Buddha Bowl:** In serving bowls, arrange cooked quinoa or brown rice, roasted sweet potatoes and chickpeas, cherry tomatoes, cucumber slices, avocado slices, and mixed greens.

4. **Drizzle with Dressing:** Drizzle the Buddha bowl with tahini dressing or your favorite dressing of choice.
5. **Garnish and Serve:** Sprinkle sesame seeds over the bowl for added texture and visual appeal. Serve with lemon wedges on the side.

Benefits:
1. **Plant-Based Protein:** Chickpeas provide plant-based protein, promoting satiety and muscle health.

2. **Vitamins and Antioxidants:** Sweet potatoes, tomatoes, cucumbers, and avocado contribute a variety of vitamins, minerals, and antioxidants.

3. **Healthy Fats:** Avocado and olive oil add heart-healthy monounsaturated fats.

4. **Fiber-Rich Grains:** Quinoa or brown rice provides dietary fiber, aiding in digestion and providing a sustained energy release.

5. **Leafy Greens:** Mixed greens offer additional vitamins, minerals, and a refreshing crunch.

Application:
- **Weeknight Dinner:** Enjoy this Buddha bowl as a quick and nutritious weeknight dinner.

- **Meal Prep:** Prepare components in advance for easy assembly throughout the week.
- **Picnic or Potluck:** Showcase this vibrant bowl at picnics or potlucks for a health-conscious and crowd-pleasing dish.

The Sweet Potato and Chickpea Buddha Bowl is a delightful and wholesome meal that brings together a variety of nutritious ingredients.

This bowl not only satisfies your taste buds but also nourishes your body with a balance of protein, fiber, and essential nutrients.

Turmeric-Ginger Chicken Soup

Scenario:
Imagine a chilly day or a moment when you need comfort and warmth. The aroma of Turmeric-Ginger Chicken Soup wafts through your kitchen, promising a bowl of nourishment and healing.

As you sip on the golden broth filled with tender chicken, vibrant vegetables, and the powerful duo of turmeric and ginger, you feel the soothing effects both on your taste buds and your well-being.

This soup is not just a meal; it's a remedy that brings comfort to your body and soul.

Ingredients:
- 1 lb boneless, skinless chicken breasts or thighs, diced
- 1 onion, finely chopped
- 3 carrots, sliced
- 3 celery stalks, sliced
- 3 cloves garlic, minced
- 1 tablespoon fresh ginger, grated
- 1 teaspoon ground turmeric
- 6 cups chicken broth (homemade or low-sodium store-bought)

- 1 cup uncooked brown rice or quinoa
- Salt and pepper to taste
- Fresh cilantro or parsley for garnish
- Lemon wedges for serving

Preparation:
1. **Sauté Aromatics:** In a large pot, sauté chopped onion, garlic, and grated ginger over medium heat until the onions are translucent and aromatic.

2. **Add Chicken:** Add diced chicken to the pot and cook until browned on all sides.

3. **Season with Turmeric:** Sprinkle ground turmeric over the chicken and vegetables. Stir well to coat the ingredients evenly.

4. **Vegetables and Rice/Quinoa:** Add sliced carrots and celery to the pot. Pour in chicken broth and bring the mixture to a boil. If using brown rice or quinoa, add it to the pot at this stage.

5. **Simmer:** Reduce the heat to low, cover the pot, and let the soup simmer for 25-30 minutes or until the chicken is cooked through, and the vegetables and grains are tender.

6. **Season and Garnish:** Season the soup with salt and pepper to taste. Garnish with fresh cilantro or parsley.

7. **Serve:** Ladle the Turmeric-Ginger Chicken Soup into bowls. Serve with lemon wedges on the side for a citrusy burst.

Benefits:
1. **Anti-Inflammatory Properties:** Turmeric contains curcumin, known for its anti-inflammatory and antioxidant properties.

2. **Digestive Aid:** Ginger is known to aid digestion and can provide relief from nausea.

3. **Lean Protein:** Chicken offers a lean source of protein, essential for muscle maintenance and repair.

4. **Nutrient-Rich Vegetables:** Carrots, celery, and onions provide essential vitamins and minerals.

5. **Whole Grains:** Brown rice or quinoa adds fiber, promoting digestive health and providing sustained energy.

Application:

- **Cold and Flu Season:** Enjoy this soup as a soothing remedy during cold and flu season for its immune-boosting properties.

- **Comfort Food:** Serve as a comforting and nourishing meal on a chilly day or when seeking solace in a bowl.

- **Meal Prep:** Prepare a batch for meal prep, as soups often taste even better the next day.

Turmeric-Ginger Chicken Soup is a delicious and healing bowl that brings together the warmth of ginger, the earthiness of turmeric, and the comfort of chicken.

It's a versatile soup that not only satisfies your taste buds but also provides a range of health benefits.

Spinach and Berry Salad

Scenario:

Imagine a sunny afternoon, and you're yearning for a refreshing and vibrant salad that captures the essence of summer. The Spinach and Berry Salad is the perfect solution.

As you toss together fresh spinach leaves, plump berries, and crunchy nuts, the colors and flavors create a symphony on your plate.

Drizzled with a tangy balsamic vinaigrette, this salad is not just a meal; it's a celebration of the season's bounty, providing a delightful blend of sweetness, crunch, and nourishment.

Ingredients:

- 6 cups fresh baby spinach leaves, washed and dried
- 1 cup strawberries, hulled and sliced
- 1 cup blueberries
- 1/2 cup raspberries
- 1/2 cup sliced almonds, toasted
- 1/4 cup crumbled feta cheese (optional)
- Balsamic vinaigrette dressing:
    - 3 tablespoons balsamic vinegar
    - 1/4 cup extra-virgin olive oil
    - 1 teaspoon Dijon mustard
    - 1 teaspoon honey or maple syrup

- Salt and pepper to taste

Preparation:

1. **Prepare Balsamic Vinaigrette:** In a small bowl, whisk together balsamic vinegar, olive oil, Dijon mustard, honey or maple syrup, salt, and pepper until well combined. Set aside.

2. **Toast Almonds:** In a dry skillet over medium heat, toast sliced almonds until golden brown and fragrant. Keep an eye on them, as they can burn quickly. Once toasted, set aside to cool.

3. **Assemble Salad:** In a large salad bowl, combine fresh baby spinach leaves, sliced strawberries, blueberries, raspberries, and toasted sliced almonds.

4. **Add Optional Feta:** If desired, sprinkle crumbled feta cheese over the salad for a savory kick.

5. **Drizzle with Dressing:** Just before serving, drizzle the balsamic vinaigrette over the salad. Toss gently to coat the ingredients evenly.

6. **Serve Immediately:** Plate the Spinach and Berry Salad on individual serving

plates or a large platter. Serve immediately to maintain the freshness and crispness of the ingredients.

Benefits:
1. **Antioxidant-Rich Berries:** Strawberries, blueberries, and raspberries are loaded with antioxidants, promoting overall health.

2. **Leafy Green Nutrients:** Spinach provides essential vitamins, minerals, and fiber for a nutritious boost.

3. **Heart-Healthy Nuts:** Toasted almonds offer healthy fats, protein, and a satisfying crunch.

4. **Optional Feta Benefits:** Feta cheese (optional) adds a creamy texture and a dose of calcium and protein.

5. **Balanced Dressing:** The balsamic vinaigrette provides a balanced blend of sweet, tangy, and savory flavors.

Application:
- **Summer Side Dish:** Serve as a refreshing side dish at summer barbecues or picnics.

- **Light Lunch:** Enjoy a generous portion as a light and satisfying lunch.

- **Impressive Starter:** Serve smaller portions as an impressive starter at dinner parties or gatherings.

Quinoa and Vegetable Stir-Fry

Scenario:

Imagine a bustling evening when you want a quick, wholesome, and flavorful dinner. The Quinoa and Vegetable Stir-Fry is the answer. As you hear the sizzle of colorful vegetables and nutty quinoa in the pan, the enticing aroma fills your kitchen.

In just a matter of minutes, you have a nutritious stir-fry that's both satisfying and packed with vibrant flavors. This dish is not just a convenient meal; it's a celebration of the goodness of fresh vegetables and protein-rich quinoa.

Ingredients:

- 1 cup quinoa, rinsed and cooked according to package instructions
- 2 tablespoons soy sauce (or tamari for a gluten-free option)
- 1 tablespoon sesame oil
- 1 tablespoon olive oil
- 2 cloves garlic, minced
- 1 tablespoon fresh ginger, grated
- 1 cup broccoli florets
- 1 bell pepper, thinly sliced (any color)
- 1 carrot, julienned

- 1 zucchini, sliced
- 1 cup snap peas, ends trimmed
- 1 cup mushrooms, sliced
- 1 cup firm tofu, cubed (optional)
- Green onions, chopped, for garnish
- Sesame seeds for garnish (optional)

Preparation:
1. **Cook Quinoa:** Rinse quinoa under cold water. In a saucepan, combine 1 cup quinoa with 2 cups water. Bring to a boil, then reduce heat to low, cover, and simmer for 15-20 minutes, or until quinoa is cooked and water is absorbed. Fluff with a fork and set aside.
2. **Prepare Stir-Fry Sauce:** In a small bowl, whisk together soy sauce and sesame oil. Set aside.

3. **Stir-Fry Vegetables:** Heat olive oil in a large wok or skillet over medium-high heat. Add minced garlic and grated ginger, and sauté for 1-2 minutes until fragrant.

4. **Add Vegetables:** Add broccoli, bell pepper, carrot, zucchini, snap peas, and mushrooms to the wok. Stir-fry for 5-7 minutes, or until the vegetables are tender-crisp.

5. **Add Tofu (Optional):** If using tofu, add cubed tofu to the vegetables and stir-fry for an additional 3-4 minutes, or until tofu is heated through.

6. **Combine Quinoa and Sauce:** Add cooked quinoa to the wok, and pour the stir-fry sauce over the mixture. Toss everything together to ensure the quinoa and vegetables are evenly coated with the sauce.

7. **Adjust Seasoning:** Taste and adjust the seasoning if needed. You can add more soy sauce or sesame oil according to your preference.

8. **Serve:** Spoon the Quinoa and Vegetable Stir-Fry onto plates or into bowls. Garnish with chopped green onions and sesame seeds if desired.

Benefits:
1. **Complete Protein Source:** Quinoa is a complete protein, providing all essential amino acids.

2. **Abundance of Vegetables:** The stir-fry is rich in a variety of vegetables, offering

a spectrum of vitamins, minerals, and antioxidants.

3. **Healthy Fats:** Sesame oil contributes healthy fats and adds a distinctive flavor.

4. **Optional Tofu Protein:** Tofu (optional) adds an extra protein boost for a more satisfying meal.

5. **Gluten-Free Option:** Tamari can be used instead of soy sauce for a gluten-free version.

Application:
- **Quick Weeknight Dinner:** Prepare this stir-fry for a quick and nutritious weeknight dinner.

- **Meal Prep:** Make a big batch for meal prep, as stir-fries are excellent for reheating.

- **Vegetarian/Vegan Option:** Enjoy as a satisfying vegetarian or vegan main dish.

Grilled Salmon with Lemon and Dill

Scenario:

Imagine a warm summer evening, and you're hosting a gathering with the tempting aroma of a sizzling grill in the air.

The centerpiece of your feast is Grilled Salmon with Lemon and Dill. As the salmon fillets cook to perfection, the combination of zesty lemon and fragrant dill creates a mouthwatering symphony of flavors.

This dish not only promises a delightful culinary experience but also showcases the simplicity and elegance of grilled salmon, making it the star of your summer soirée.

Ingredients:
- 4 salmon fillets, skin-on
- 2 tablespoons olive oil
- Zest of 1 lemon
- Juice of 1 lemon
- 2 tablespoons fresh dill, chopped
- Salt and black pepper to taste
- Lemon slices for garnish
- Fresh dill sprigs for garnish

Preparation:

1. **Prepare the Marinade:** In a bowl, whisk together olive oil, lemon zest, lemon juice, chopped dill, salt, and black pepper.

2. **Marinate the Salmon:** Place the salmon fillets in a shallow dish or a resealable plastic bag. Pour the marinade over the fillets, ensuring they are well-coated. Marinate in the refrigerator for at least 30 minutes, allowing the flavors to infuse.

3. **Preheat the Grill:** Preheat your grill to medium-high heat. Make sure the grates are clean and lightly oiled to prevent sticking.

4. **Grill the Salmon:** Remove the salmon from the marinade and place the fillets on the preheated grill, skin side down. Grill for about 4-5 minutes per side or until the salmon easily flakes with a fork. Cooking times may vary based on the thickness of the fillets.

5. **Baste with Marinade:** While grilling, baste the salmon with some of the remaining marinade using a brush. This adds extra flavor and helps keep the salmon moist.

6. **Garnish and Serve:** Once the salmon is cooked through, transfer it to a serving platter. Garnish with lemon slices and fresh dill sprigs.

7. **Serve Immediately:** Serve the Grilled Salmon with Lemon and Dill immediately, allowing your guests to enjoy the salmon while it's warm and flavorful.

Benefits:
1. **Rich in Omega-3 Fatty Acids:** Salmon is a rich source of omega-3 fatty acids, which are beneficial for heart health.

2. **Lean Protein:** Salmon provides high-quality protein, essential for muscle maintenance and repair.

3. **Vitamin D:** Salmon is a natural source of vitamin D, crucial for bone health and immune function.

4. **Antioxidant-Rich Lemon and Dill:** Lemon provides vitamin C, while dill offers antioxidants and adds a fresh, aromatic flavor.

5. **Heart-Healthy Olive Oil:** The use of olive oil contributes monounsaturated fats, supporting heart health.

Application:

- **Summer BBQs:** Feature Grilled Salmon with Lemon and Dill as a star attraction at summer barbecues.

- **Family Dinners:** Serve this dish for a special family dinner, impressing your loved ones with a delicious and healthy main course.

- **Entertaining Guests:** Impress your guests at dinner parties with this elegant yet straightforward grilled salmon recipe.

CONCLUSION

As you finish the "Eat Well, Live Well Cookbook," we hope you've had a shift in how you see and connect with the food on your table, not merely a culinary excursion.

This cookbook is more than just a compilation of recipes; it's a monument to the notion that living a healthy lifestyle is a never-ending, delectable adventure.

We hope that these pages have inspired you to think of your kitchen as a place for creativity, sustenance, and self-care. Eating healthily is a journey, not a destination, and we urge you to apply what you've learned here to your everyday culinary endeavors.

May the vivid tastes, nutritional ingredients, and culinary knowledge given in these recipes accompany you on your journey toward a life that balances wellness and enjoyment.

May you discover delight in the process of making meals that nourish not just the body but also the spirit as you continue to relish each mouthful.

Thank you for include the "Eat Well, Live Well Cookbook" in your culinary adventure. Here's to a future full of tasty discoveries, conscious decisions, and a celebration of the limitless advantages of eating well and living well. Cheers to a life full of taste and vigor, as well as the simple pleasures found on a well-balanced plate.